Contents

Dedication	3
Copyright	4
1. Are You Prepared For This?	5
2. Superficial or 1ST Degree Burns	6
Extent of Burn	*7*
Please Remember!	8
Description of 1st Degree Burns	*8*
3. Partial Thickness or 2ND Degree Burn	10
4. Full Thickness or 3RD Degree Burn	12
Full Thickness Burns in the Facial Area.	*12*
Full Thickness Burns of the Hand	*13*
Other Areas	*14*
5. Skin Grafts	15
Organic Materials May Include—	*15*
6. Scar Therapy	18
Keloid Scars	*18*
Hypertrophic Scars	*19*
Elasticized Pressure Garment	*21*
7. Psychological Effects of Burns Scarring	22
8. MRSA (Golden Staph)	23
9. Burns First Aid	25
Superficial Burns First Aid	*25*
Partial Thickness Burns First Aid	*25*
Full Thickness Burns First Aid	*26*
Before you are faced with a Burns Accident	*27*
Consider these as Essential Items	*28*
Optional items	*29*
10. Pain & Pain Management	30
Pain Medications	*31*
Interventional procedures	*32*
About the Author	34

Table of Illustrations

Superficial burn 9
Partial thickness burn 11
Full thickness burn 13
Left hand completely healed 14
Dermatome harvesting split skin 16
Split skin after meshing 16
Meshed skin applied to wound 17
Prototype skin spray device... 20
Hypertrophic Scarring.. 21
Scar contractures... 24
A bad case of sunburn 27
Author Pete and Wife Aileen on Hong Kong Holiday two years after discharge from the Burns Ward... 34

Dedication

To my wife, Aileen, and kids, who bore the brunt of my pain!

Copyright

© 2014 by Robert P Rumball

All rights reserved. No part of this document may be reproduced or transmitted in any form or by any means, electronic, mechanical, photocopying, recording or otherwise, without prior written permission of Robert P Rumball.

1. Are You Prepared For This?

Suddenly, I was burning from the waist up, the flames roaring around my ears.

In a blind panic I started to run, but that made the flames roar louder, I was on steeply sloping ground covered with long grass, so I started to roll in the grass until I found myself under the nearby house, and the flames were licking at the floor boards, and I had to get out. I remember thinking that I wouldn't want to burn the house down as well.

A scary picture? Sure it is, and a true one that happened to me over 30 years ago.

How many people would know the correct thing to do if they were suddenly faced with an accident like this...Would you?

Let's follow the story a bit more...

Crawling up the hill, still burning, somebody had got the garden hose and watered me down, and kept the hose running on me, not only putting the putting the fire out, but the prolonged running of cool water was an absolute relief.

Bloody hell! It felt good!

And I do remember that feeling of relief even more clearly than the shock of finding myself burning. But back to the story...

By this time a fair crowd had gathered, but I wasn't really aware of anything excepting the long treacly skeins of melted skin sliding off my hand and arm.

The amazing thing that dawned on me THEN, was, there was absolutely NO PAIN!

But that didn't last very long, by the time our family doctor got there, the pain had become horrendous, and the shot of some sort of painkiller that he gave me was a godsend.

OK! That's enough of that; except to say that my burns were calculated at sixty per cent, with about half that area being a full thickness, or third degree burn, and the rest, partial thickness or second degree burns.

My purpose in writing this book is to get people to think about their own reactions if they were ever faced with a burns accident, which usually results in the most painful injuries possible, so we'll skip the next 3 months in the Burns Ward of the Royal Brisbane Hospital, and the several skin grafts which happened whilst there.

Think about this point. If you are faced with something like this, it would more than likely be one of your immediate family involved.

As I found out much later, the prompt running of cool water over me from the garden hose was simply the best thing that could have been done for me. Apart from putting the fire out, and giving me such blessed relief, it achieved something vitally important for the future outcome of my burns.

The cooling water stopped the burn from penetrating deeper.

My burn was from gasoline, and that type of burn can continue to penetrate human tissue for up to 17 minutes, so who knows how much more full thickness burn would have occurred, had the cool water not been applied for at least half an hour?

Let's look at the degrees of Burn Thickness.

2. Superficial or 1st Degree Burns

Superficial Burns are those which only affect the Epidermis. Sunburn is a typical example.

What does burn thickness mean? What difference does it make?

Burn thickness is important because the different layers of the skin all have many different functions. Your skin protects and insulates you. It can grow new skin, regulate body temperature, grow hair, guard against infection and communicate with your brain about what your environment feels like. The supple flexibility of your skin allows you to move and breath.

How deep a burn penetrates through the layers of the skin determines which of these functions may be damaged and which of these functions may be lost forever. A close inspection of the texture, moisture, color and general appearance of a burn will give you important clues regarding what thickness or "degree" of burn the patient has suffered.

It is not important, at this stage, to try to estimate the extent of the burn. But it is vitally important to COOL IT, with cool water, not cold, applied gently, and to not attempt to remove any clothing.

Extent of Burn

In Calculating the Percentage of Body Surface area that has been affected by burns, the following guide is universally used.

- For smaller burns, the palm of the patient's hand is 1%, not including the fingers.
- The head is 9%.
- The chest and back are both 18% respectively.
- Each leg is also 18%.
- Each arm is given 9%
- The genitalia add the remaining 1% to total body area.

From that foundation, large area burns can be estimated rapidly, for example:
One half of one arm is a 4.5% of TBSA (Total Body Surface Area). One entire leg and the front of the other leg is a 27% of TBSA burn.

Please Remember!

This is Vitally Important!

Prompt cooling of the burn can prevent a second degree burn from escalating to a Full Thickness Burn.

A burn from Gasoline can continue to penetrate tissue for up to 17 minutes.

So continue to cool the area for at least 20 minutes, but no longer, as it may reduce the blood supply to the injury.

Only ever use <u>COOL</u> water, applied gently, **never** use Cold Water, and do not attempt to remove clothing.

If water from a hose is not available, use any container filled with water and apply using soaked hand towels.

Description of 1st Degree Burns

Superficial burns such as sunburn showing redness, slight swelling and mild pain can be safely handled by home treatment if the burnt area is less than 50% of the body surface.

- These burns involve only the uppermost layer of the skin, also known as the epidermis. The epidermis is a thin layer of cells that coat the outer surface of the body. This thin coating of cells is what we traditionally think of when we reference the skin.
- The epidermis functions primarily as a protective layer. It protects us from infection and UV rays.
- Burns of the epidermis are red and painful. They do not tend to blister. Blisters are the first sign of damage to the dermal layer below the epidermis. Contact burns that redden and hurt but do not blister are also classified as 1st Degree Burns.

After the initial cooling of a contact burn, or for Sunburn treatment, a Burn Cream or Aloe Vera can be applied to keep the air currents from causing pain.

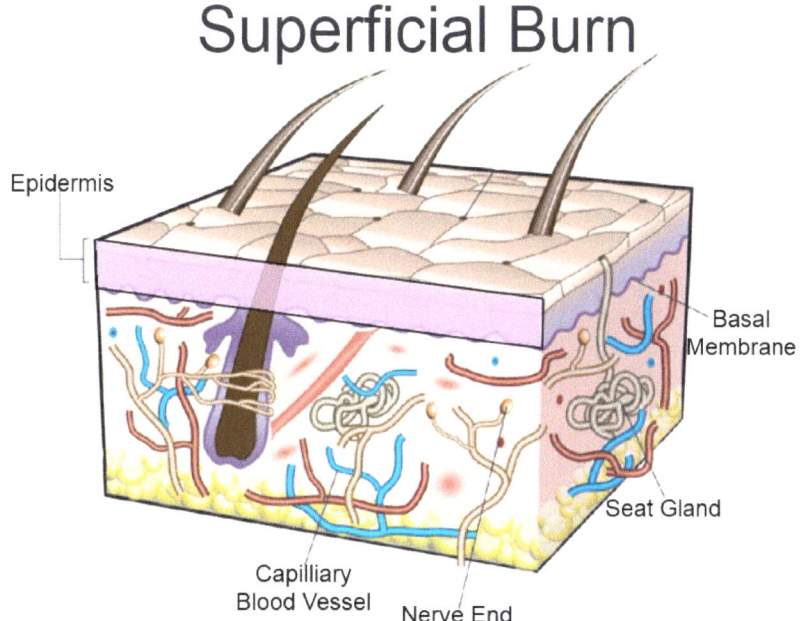

3. Partial Thickness or 2nd Degree Burn

Partial thickness burns don't extend completely through the dermis. As you can see, these burns although very painful, usually heal well and are easier to care for. This is because new skin can grow upward from the dermis.

The patient should see a physician if,
- More than 1% of skin surface is involved (more than the size of the patient's palm).
- Face, neck, genital area, hands, or feet are involved.
- Any child under 12 suffering from burns or scalds.
- Description of Partial Thickness Burns
- Second Degree Burns penetrate into the dermal layer. The epidermis is destroyed and the dermis is damaged to varying degrees but the underlying subcutaneous issues remain undamaged.
- The dermis is a fluid rich layer beneath the epidermis. Within the dermis lay our nerve endings, pores, hair follicles and cells responsible for the growth and regeneration of skin. Depending on the depth of involvement, all of these functions are at risk.
- Without the intact epidermis, the skin tissues are no longer protected from UV light and, more importantly, bacteria. Partial and full thickness burns are at great risk for infection, hence the use of Silver Sulfadiazine on these deeper burns. It was used on me 30 odd year ago and is still in use today.
- Depending on the extent of dermal damage the patient may also lose the ability to sweat and, therefore, cool the body. This is the only lasting legacy that I have from my burns. The left arm cannot sweat, nor can my left ribcage, both of which are important to the body's cooling system.

It would be a bit like a car with half the radiator blocked up with grass seeds and grasshoppers. it would run hot, as I do.

- If nerve endings are destroyed the patient will lose feeling in the region. Hair may no longer grow within the damaged area and if growth cells are destroyed, the skin will lose its ability to regenerate and heal.
- Patients with second degree burns are at danger for losing some of the mobility in the body region affected.
- Partial thickness burns may be covered by the destroyed epidermal layer or open. If skin covers the burn it will be grey, wrinkled or blistered. Open burns will be red or white and appear moist

Deeper partial thickness burns will scar, and show as a slightly raised patch, and because the Melanin cells have been destroyed or damaged, that area will have no pigmentation, and be very susceptible to sunburn.

Partial Thickness Burn

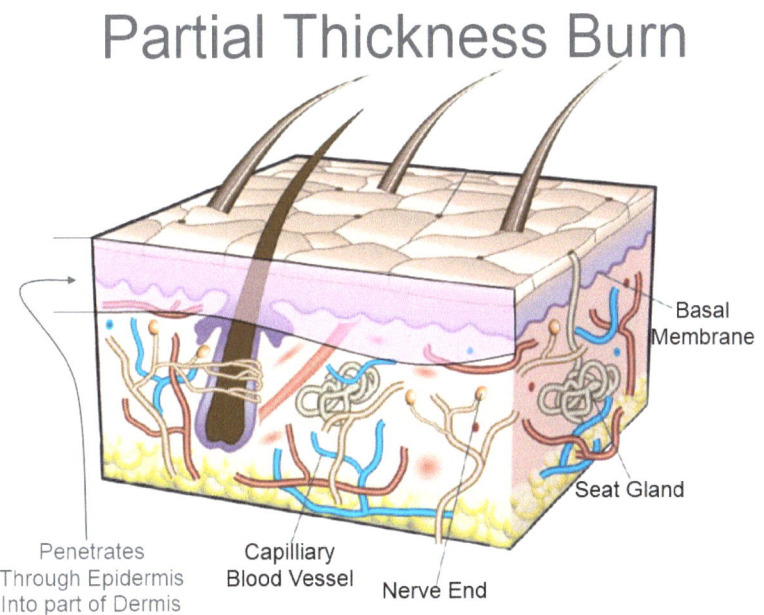

4. Full Thickness or 3rd Degree Burn

If the Dermis is destroyed, no skin can grow back in that area and deep scarring develops unless Skin Grafting is performed. These burns appear white or blackened and because the nerves have been destroyed, the patient will have no pain in the affected area.

You should never self-treat a full thickness burn, no matter how small. The risk of infection and scarring is too high.

Do Not attempt to remove clothing that may be stuck to the wound.

Full thickness burns penetrate completely through the epidermal and dermal layer. All epidermal and dermal functions are lost at the burn area. These burns can enter the subcutaneous fat layer and occasionally the muscle or bone. (Then called a 4th degree burn)

Full thickness burns appear waxy and dry. They will be white, brown or black and appear charred. The patient will not experience pain at the site of the full thickness but will likely feel intense pain in the partial thickness burn areas around the full thickness site.

Full Thickness Burns in the Facial Area.

The face houses all 5 senses, and can produce a complex array of emotional signals. More than any other feature, the face is responsible for how the world views each of us and, in turn, how we interpret our world. Because of these distinctions, care and management of the burned face is important both psychologically, and cosmetically.

Unlike deep burns elsewhere, facial burns are mostly handled conservatively, and when possible, are treated open, with ointments. The infection of facial wounds is uncommon, allowing treatment to be concentrated on conservation of vital tissue.

If some areas do need resurfacing, careful spot grafting is performed using Full Thickness, or Thicker Split-skin (approx.38mm) Autograft to prevent scar contractures.

Full Thickness Burns of the Hand

The care and management of hand burns is almost as important as it is for facial burns. The palm is usually spared due to involuntary fist clenching at the time of burning, but when the palm suffers deep burns, the wounds have a poor prognosis

In full thickness burns of the back of the hand, early skin grafting is desirable as long as aggressive physiotherapy is started early. My left hand was completely 'De-Gloved', but apart from the inside finger areas, the thicker than usual skin of my palm saved my palm from 3rd degree burns. The entire back of the hand was covered with split skin graft sheet, as was my arm right up to the elbow. Physiotherapy on my fingers was started very early and seemed to last a couple of hours per day for several days; it was so easy to doze off while the Physiotherapist worked on each finger. It was highly successful and it wasn't long after that I could 'make a fist' by clenching my fingers.

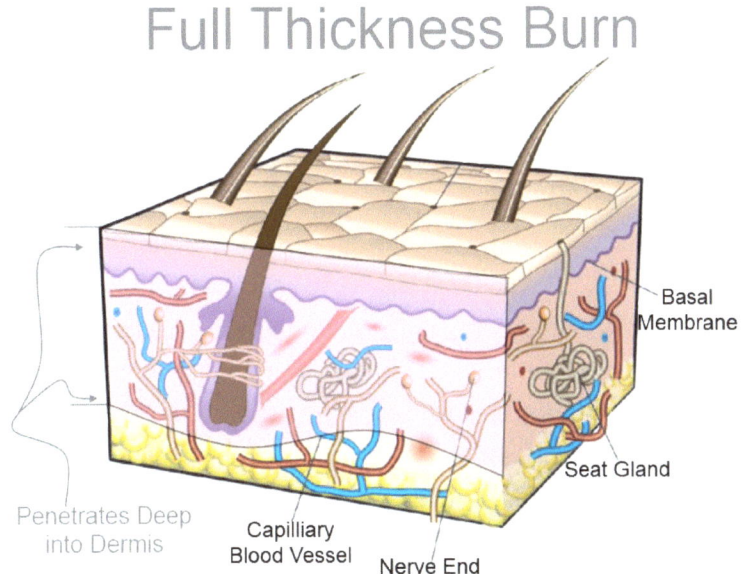

Since then I have had full use of that hand, excepting for the over-all loss of feeling, mainly in my fingertips which precluded me from carrying on with any manually demanding pursuits.

I was very lucky in that a visiting surgeon did this job, and that he had the expertise to spare my dorsal hand veins and tendons, and to position all finger joints in full flexion prior to graft application.

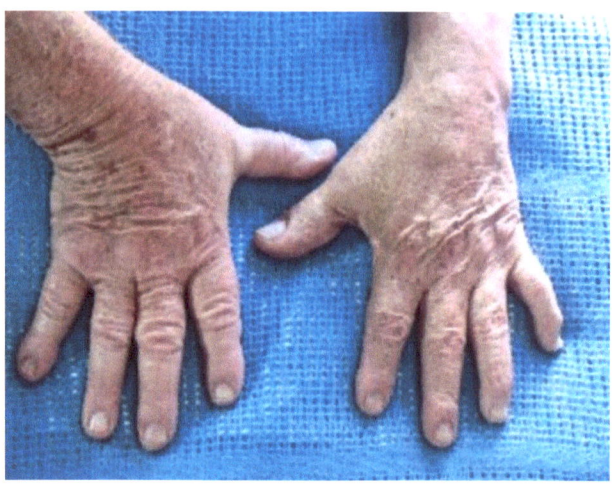

Other Areas

Burns of the perineum are unusual with major burn injuries. Many perineal burns will heal by contraction if kept clean, Colostomy is not necessary. Burns of the penis may cause more problems secondary to contracture. Penile full-thickness burn may be conservatively debrided and grafted to minimize contractures.

Revisions following grafting for penile burns are frequent. In women, burns involving the breasts have important psychological and cosmetic implications. Sheet grafts are preferred for coverage.

Nipple burns will often repair naturally from the lactiferous ducts, and conservative management is indicated. Full thickness burns debriding and resurfacing, involving the trunk in young females most often spare the breast bud, which should not be included in the excision specimen. Scars constrict growth and hinder development.

5. Skin Grafts

Treating Burns with Antimicrobial dressings can adversely affect wound healing, and they require daily maintenance, whereas Biological dressings have no direct toxins or antimicrobial properties.

However, they do reduce loss of heat, water, protein and red blood cells, and promote more rapid wound healing.

Biological dressings also reduce burn wound pain.

These materials may be organic or synthetic in origin, but good wound adherence especially in 3rd degree burns is the key function.

Organic Materials May Include—

Autograft is usually only possible if the patient's burns are less than 70%, otherwise the other alternatives for treating burns would be checked.

Autografts are taken from the thighs or buttocks where the resulting scars would be hidden. The thickness of the skin used takes in the Epidermis and part of the Dermis, about the equivalent of 2nd Degree Burns; it is then put through a meshing machine which allows the skin to be expanded from 2 to 4 times its original area.

Healing of subsequent skin where Autograft has been used can be expected in areas of good allograft 'take', thereby eliminating hypertrophic scarring.

Fresh skin allograft has become the standard for temporary coverage of the clean open burn wound; it achieves an environmental 'seal' of the burn wound at the graft-wound interface and improves the host's immune defences.

The illustration below shows a Dermatome being used to harvest split skin from a thigh. The skin will then be put through a Meshing machine to increase the coverage.

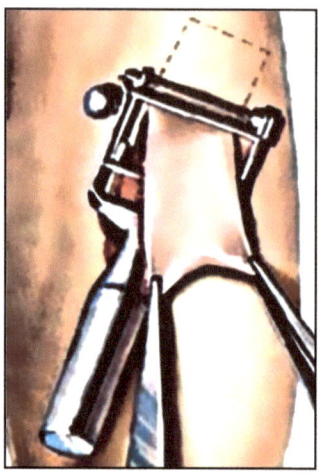

Below: Illustration of 'Meshed' skin. After healing, the area will show tiny, almost invisible, scars in the open parts of the mesh, but the healing will be accelerated.

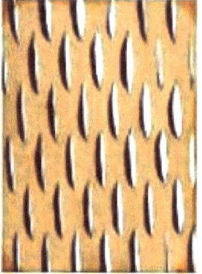 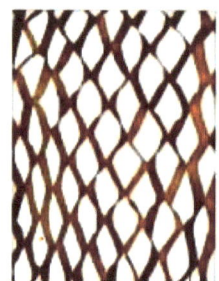

Below: Meshed Split Skin being applied to wound.

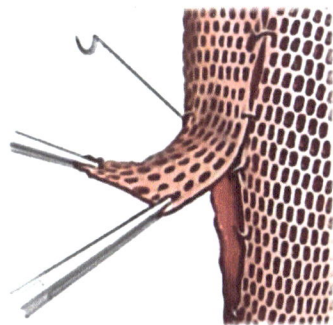

Homograft human skin graft can be obtained from fresh cadavers within 18 hours of death. The graft can re-vascularize once adhered to the wound, but rejection will occur within 14 days.

I had a strip of Homograft across the upper chest area, and it did try to remain part of me, but after a couple of weeks became very smelly.

When it was peeled off, the healing underneath was incredible, and now only faint scarring is visible.

Xenograft (pigskin) degenerates before it is rejected but provides the same level of protection from infection as allograft, so pigskin is often embedded with salts of antimicrobial agents to increase its bacteriostatic potential. Pigskin is cheaper and more available than allograft. Its recommended uses include protective coverage of partial-thickness wounds and should be changed every 3-4 days to prevent infection.

Artificial Skin dressings provide wound protection, increase the rate of wound healing, and reduce patient discomfort. Very careful application is essential.

When used to cover clean partial-thickness wounds, the dressing detaches as healing occurs underneath.

Biobrane© is a synthetic, membrane with an outer silicone layer bonded to an inner collagen nylon matrix. Its elasticity and transparency allows easy drape ability, fuller range of movement and easy wound inspection. The major problems with Biobrane© in treating burns are its expense and its lack of inherent antimicrobial properties. Wound infections are not uncommon.

6. Scar Therapy

Scar Therapy and removal treatments are often expensive and invasive, and are only relevant for deep 2nd Degree Burns or 3rd Degree Burns that leave disfiguring or disabling Scar Contractures.

The main concerns are:

Keloid Scars

These are a more serious form of burns scarring, because they can carry on growing indefinitely into a large, tumorous (although benign) neoplasm.

Keloids can occur on anyone, but they are most common in dark-skinned people, and can be caused by surgery, an accident, by acne or, sometimes, from body piercings.

Although they can be a cosmetic problem, keloids are only inert masses of collagen and therefore completely harmless and non-cancerous, but they can be itchy or painful in some individuals, tending to be most common on the shoulders and chest.

One way that keloids are treated is through steroids. In this case, doctors will inject steroid drugs into the skin around the keloid. Keloid treatment using steroids requires the patient to visit a doctor multiple times for the injections.

Although steroids have been successful, it should be noted that patients with darker skin can suffer from tissue atrophy or hypopigmentation, the loss of skin color.

Patients who choose to treat their scars through steroids are often given shots of the steroid hydrocortisone every two to three weeks.

Excision is also a viable alternative method of keloid treatment, and requires the surgical removal of all the scar tissue. Excisions are not always successful, and in some cases the keloid reoccurs after the tissue has been removed and begins to heal again.

Treating keloids can be very frustrating for patients, and methods are still being researched. There are no definitive cure-alls currently available for those battling the scars.

Dermatologists and plastic surgeons are still exploring ways to both prevent and treat keloids. One of the newest advancements in keloid therapy is the use of lasers to decrease the size of the keloid and improve the color of the scar.

Hypertrophic Scars

Are often distinguished from keloids by their lack of growth outside the original wound area.

Hypertrophic scars occur when the body overproduces collagen, which causes an area of fibrous tissue to replace normal skin and is a natural part of the healing process.

These scars take the form of a red raised ridge or lump on the skin and do not grow outside the wound area, and are not as prominent as Keloid scars.

They are also minimised by the use of a pressure garment.

A recently developed Spray-on Skin Cells process invented by Dr Fiona Wood, head of the Royal Perth Hospital Burns Department shows great promise in the treatment of extensive full thickness burns, which will greatly reduce the occurrence of scarring in burns patients.

In 1992 a schoolteacher was admitted to the hospital with petrol burns to 90% of his body and Dr Wood used the newly invented US technology of Cultured Skin to save his life.

Working with a scientist, Marie Stoner, they moved from growing sheets of skin to producing spray-able skin cells, and gained worldwide acclaim.

Dr Wood had found that burns scarring is greatly reduced if covering skin can be provided within 10 days.

Previous techniques needed 3 weeks to produce enough material to cover major burns, but Dr Wood has reduced that to five days by culturing small biopsies into larger volumes of skin cell suspensions.

Below: Prototype Skin Spray Device

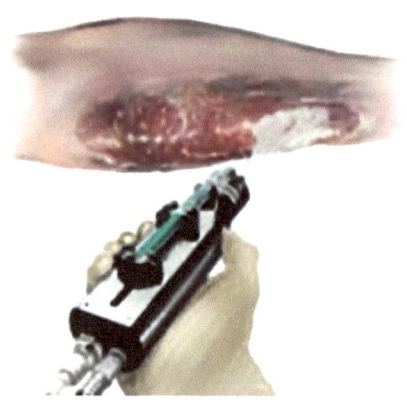

Below: Typical Hypertrophic Scar

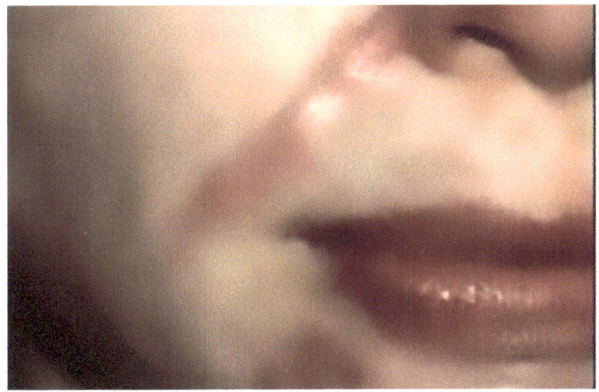

Elasticized Pressure Garment

My 'Jobst' pressure suit was fitted, after careful measuring, from my knees to the top of my head, and including my left arm and hand.

This is about the time that the really serious ITCHING begins as the body sends out heaps of Histamine to aid the healing process. Anti-Histamine tablets help keep it under control... a bit, also Aloe Vera liquid helped to moisturise the skin, soften the scars and allow the pressure garment to do its job more easily.

Wearing the pressure garment for the first time is difficult because of the discomfort, and the inability to scratch the healing wounds. But you soon learn to slide a pencil or ruler down inside the elasticised suit to scratch the itchy spot.

After few days of continual wearing, it becomes a part of you, and when you remove it for bathing, you feel as if your body is falling apart, literally, and you can't wait to put it back on.

I wore the entire suit 24/7 for over a year, and then continued with the glove and arm-piece for another 6 months with the result that the scars on my arm and hand flattened out completely.

7. Psychological Effects of Burns Scarring

The excruciating pain of a burns accident, followed by the usually painful treatment of severe burns, often produces psychopathological responses, which, when combined with the long-term disfiguring effects of burns scarring can lead to depression and post-traumatic stress disorder (PTSD).

Patients at risk of depression are those who suffered depression pre-burn, and females, together with facial or obvious scarring.

PTSD risk factors are pre-burn depression, type and seriousness of the injury, fearfulness related to pain, and the visibility of the burns injury.

Looking back at it now I find all that hard to believe, and it was not until my wife reminded me, that I did remember those feelings, including my sensitivity relating to my burns scarring.

The hardest thing that I had to face at this time was my daughter's wedding, about 4 months after leaving the Burns Ward. The reception was held in the Golf Club, and we had some 200 guests. I got through my speech OK and even managed a couple of jokes, but was so very conscious of my appearance. My scarlet face was a stark contrast to my mid-blue coat.

From the extensive research that I've done on this subject, I've found that Psychological and Psychopathology problems are considered to exist in a 'Significant Minority' of burns patients, and that post-burn screening of 'Mood and Anxiety Disorders' should be carried out, and treated, if indicated.

I have no doubt now, looking back, and considering my new-found knowledge, that I was certainly affected by some psychological problems, but would never have accepted that then, and most certainly would not have accepted 'Counseling', always having been a sceptic on that topic.

8. MRSA (Golden Staph)

The Long Name is methicillin-resistant Staphylococcus aureus, which is a type of Staphylococcus aureus (Golden Staph) that is resistant to methicillin and other related antibiotics of the penicillin class, is commonly found on the skin and/or in the noses of healthy people.

Penicillin revolutionised the treatment of Staphylococcus aureus in the 1940's, however the ability of the Golden Staph to negate Penicillin's efficiency led to most strains of Staphylococcus aureus becoming resistant by 1960.

A new type of penicillin antibiotic called methicillin was developed early in 1960 and proved effective, and then newer and more effective drugs were developed such as flucloxacillin.

Eventually Staphylococcus aureus developed a resistance to flucloxacillin and Methicillin, becoming known as "methicillin-resistant Staphylococcus aureus".

There are other antibiotics which can be used to treat these infections, but these are not generally available in tablet form, and must be administered by drip or injection.

Methicillin-resistant Staphylococcus aureus is usually harmless until it gets into the body through an open wound. It can cause havoc in a Hospital burns ward where wounds are open to the air for therapeutic reasons.

Similar to Golden Staph, the resistant strain can colonise on the skin or inside the nose of a patient who then becomes a virtual reservoir.

Hospital staff are regularly checked by having a nose swab taken, and if found to be positive, they get a few days off to eradicate it.

In the home environment it can be so easily wiped out by observing due diligence to cleanliness.

Methicillin-resistant Staphylococcus aureus can exist on inanimate objects, so before entering or leaving a hospital ward, it is imperative that hands are cleaned by using the supplied cleanser.

Surgical Wards have a much stricter regime, requiring disposable gowns, caps and gloves to be worn.

At this point I must mention how I was discharged from the burns ward after 3 months, but a few weeks early because the ward had to be closed down so that they could eradicate the MRSA that had taken over.

My left side had an open wound about the size of a small dinner plate where the Split-Skin grafts would not take because I was still infected with the "MRSA Bug". My wife, Aileen received a crash course in wound and MRSA management, and she took me home. I was very weak, but very pleased to be going home.

After 2 weeks at home with Aileen doing all the wound dressings twice a day, I had to return to the burns ward for further treatment.

Lo and Behold! A test for MRSA came back negative, and the huge wound had shrunk to a mere hand-span.

So they sent me home again.

This shows how MRSA can be beaten in a domestic environment provided that normal hygiene precautions are observed.

Below: Scar Contractures.

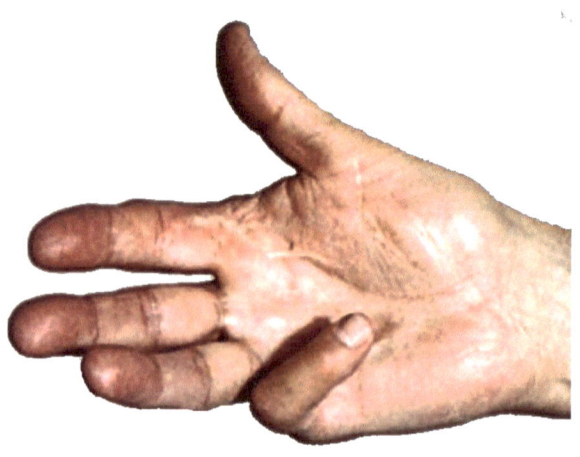

9. Burns First Aid

When first confronted with a burns victim, the prime consideration, after removing him/her from the danger area, should be the immediate cooling of the burns (Never Use Cold Water), even before attempting to determine the Depth or Extent of the injury.

Superficial Burns First Aid

Burn first aid involves cooling the outermost layer of the skin (Epidermis). This layer keeps all the body fluids in, and keeps bacteria outside the body from entering. In a superficial burn the epidermis has not been injured very badly, and is considered a minor burn unless sensitive areas such as the face, groin, buttocks, or the hands and feet are affected.

- Firstly get the patient away from the source of heat.

- Run cool water over the burn or place a cool compress over it, this cools the burn, prevents swelling, and helps to relieve pain.

- Apply soothing Burn Cream or **Aloe Vera Gel** to the site.

Partial Thickness Burns First Aid

This has penetrated down into the dermis. A layer of fluid collects between the epidermis and the dermis, which causes blistering. 2nd degree burns show swelling and are extremely painful.

- Remove the patient from the source of the burn.

- Run water over the burn or place moist towels over the burn to reduce the swelling and cool the burn. If the burn is larger than a hand-span treat it as a major burn, especially if it's on the face, hands, feet, buttocks, groin or major joint. Large second degree burns should be treated like an emergency. Dial Emergency and get medical help immediately.

Full Thickness Burns First Aid

Usually painless because the nerve endings have been burned away and the difficulty is in knowing just how severe the burns might be. The burn will have penetrated right down to the fatty layer, and perhaps even deeper, to the muscle layers and even to the bone. The burn first aid should involve------

- Get the patient away from the source of the burn

- As soon as possible gently run cool water over the burns for at least 20 minutes

- .Call the Emergency Number for your location

- The victim should be lying down with feet elevated above the heart to prevent the symptoms of shock.

- Cool moist towels should be placed over the burns.

- DO NOT try to remove clothing that is stuck to a burned area.

- When Emergency Services arrive, **keep out of the way**.

Before you are faced with a Burns Accident

You really need to **regularly** check out your First Aid Kit to make sure that any perishable items are still inside the Use-By Date.

Very few First Aid Kits deal with even a Minor Burns Injury.

Major Burns Injuries on a large scale are another matter of course, but I would bet that there aren't many families around who haven't had at least a minor burn to cope with.

And of course the most common is **SUNBURN**.

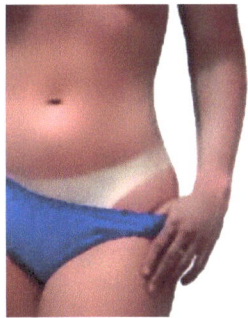

The trouble is that most products for treating minor burns do have a limited shelf life, and cannot be included in the list of items as advertised by the companies supplying the kits.

As a 3rd Degree Burns Survivor, and also one who suffered blistering sunburn as a child, I feel compelled to offer a page or two on First Aid Kits.

Consider these as Essential Items

For a General Purpose Kit:

- At least nine sterile, cotton-gauze swabs, for cleaning wounds and placing over non-adherent burn dressings.

- At least three disposable hand towels or tissues, for general cleaning, other than wounds.

- 24 sterile, adhesive dressing strips in assorted widths, to cover small cuts, blisters and abrasions.

- One roll of low-allergenic adhesive strapping, at least 25mm wide x 2.5m long, to hold dressings in place.

- Two sterile, individually packed, non-adhesive dry dressings, 100 x 100mm, to use for burns, abrasions, cuts, lacerations and weeping wounds.

- Three sterile wound dressings of different sizes, to protect wounds, use as an eye-pad, or help control bleeding by applying pressure.

- Three rolls of stretch bandage, 50, 75 and 100mm wide and at least 1.5m long (and stretchable to twice that length), to hold dressings in place, support injured limbs or give first aid for poisonous bites.

- Two triangular calico bandages with at least 900 mm edge length each, to use as slings or dressings, or as bandages to hold large dressings or splints in place.

- At least five safety pins about 40mm long, to hold bandages in place.

- One pair of rust-resistant scissors about 100mm long, with at least one blunt point, to cut dressings and bandages, or to cut away clothing.

- One pair of rust-resistant pointed forceps, with accurately aligned tips and in a protective case, for removing splinters and stings.

- One pencil and notepad, to record times and details or for passing messages.

- At least three sealable plastic bags, about 150 x 200mm, for carrying water, making ice packs, disposing of dirty dressings or carrying severed body parts.

- Disposable latex gloves and an approved resuscitation mask, for infection control.

- First aid information — books are available from expert ambulance services.

Optional items

- At least six individually wrapped isopropyl alcohol swabs, for cleaning areas around wounds.

- One sterile, thick and absorbent 'combine' dressing, 90 x 200mm, to cover wounds.

- One plastic squeeze-bottle of saline solution, about 100ml, clearly labelled with usage instructions and expiry date, to clean eyes, wounds and burns.

- One aluminium foil blanket, to keep a casualty warm.

- Sting relief treatment, 10ml minimum, clearly labelled with its purpose and expiry date, to relieve discomfort from stings or bites.

- Hydrogel burn treatment, to treat burns if no cool water is available.

- Aloe Vera Gel, about 100ml, clearly labelled with usage instructions and expiry date, to apply to superficial burns, sunburn.

- Proprietary brand of Burn Cream with painkilling ability, usage instructions and expiry date.

- Fire Blanket, should be in every household, not as part of the Kit, but essential for putting out a fire on the stove-top or on a person. If anyone of your family works on motors, or uses inflammables for an occupation or hobby, I would regard a Fire Blanket as mandatory.

The last five items are my additions to a recommendation by Choice Magazine for a First Aid Kit, and apart from the Fire Blanket, would not impose much of a burden physically or financially.

10. Pain & Pain Management

Pain can be Short Term, as caused by an underlying trauma or disease, which is eased once healing occurs, and/or treated with drugs. Effective Long Term Pain Management, however, often demands Pharmacologic measures, Physical Therapy, Interventional procedures, and Psychological measures, either individually or in various combinations.

- Acute pain medication is for rapid onset of pain such as from an inflicted Trauma or from Post-operative pain.
- Chronic pain medication is for alleviating long-lasting, ongoing pain.

Pain Medications

It is beyond the scope of this report to discuss the various types of drugs that are used to treat pain, as the following generic groups each contain so many types, the lists growing constantly.

- Non-Steroidal Anti Inflammatory Drugs (NSAID) generally have a limited effect in Chronic pain treatment due to the adverse effects of long-term use.
- Opioids

Can provide a short, intermediate or long acting pain relief, depending upon the specific properties of the medication, and whether it is produced as an extended release drug.

- Antidepressants and Anti-epileptic drugs.

These drugs are often prescribed 'Off-Label' for chronic pain management and act mainly within the pain pathways of the central nervous system.

They are generally more effective in treating neuropathic pain disorders, and have a longer list of side effects than opiate or NSAID treatments for chronic pain, and including the risk of seizures resulting from suddenly ceasing Anti-epileptics.

Interventional procedures

Typically used for Chronic Back pain, include Epidural Steroid Injections, Neurolytic Blocks, Facet Joint Injections, Spinal Cord Stimulators, and Intrathecal Implants.

The number of Interventional Procedures for pain has grown over the last few years.

- Physical Therapy is either used alone or simultaneously with Pharmacologic measures, Interventional procedures, and Behavioural Therapy to treat pain, usually as part of a multidisciplinary program.

- Acupuncture has shown effectiveness for the treatment of pain, and, in some cases of acute pain in the abdomen area, face, headache, knee, low back, neck, dentistry and sciatica.

Further proof is needed for claims of effectiveness in other conditions because trials originating in China are all positive (not as a result of Fraud, but of publication bias), whereas trials in the West show a mixture of positive, negative and neutral results.

- Cognitive and Behavioural Therapy using stress reduction and relaxation has been found to reduce chronic pain in some patients, although a large number of patients gain no benefit.

- Hypnosis was reviewed in 2007, which found evidence for its effectiveness in the reduction of pain in some conditions, although the trial only included 13 cases. The report concluded that a lot more research would be needed.

Inadequate treatment of pain is common in all departments; in the management of all forms of chronic pain including cancer pain, and in end of life care.

The World Health Organization (WHO) estimated in late 2008 that about 80 per cent of the world population has either no or inadequate access to treatment for moderate to severe pain. Yet the pain treatment medications are cheap, safe, effective, relatively uncomplicated to administer, and international law obliges countries to make adequate pain medications available.

Reasons for under-treatment in pain management include cultural, societal, religious, and political attitudes. Furthermore, the physicians concentrate on the physical aspects of the trauma or disease rather than quality of life.

Other reasons may have to do with inadequate training, personal biases or fear of prescription drug abuse and fear of being accused of over-prescribing.

Current strategies being applied for improved pain management include, drawing it up as an ethical issue, advancing it as a legal right, classifying failure to provide pain management as professional misconduct, and publishing guidelines and standards of practice by professional bodies.

About the Author

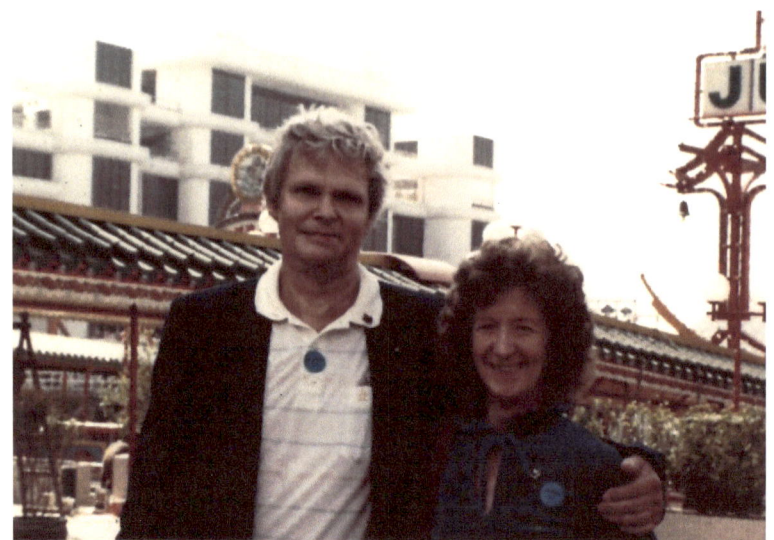

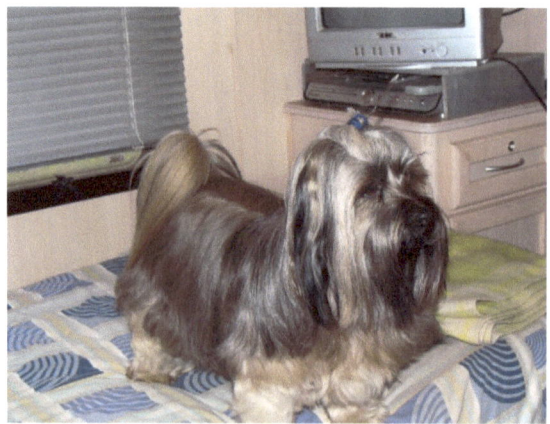

Pete and Aileen on holiday in Hong Kong two years after his discharge from the Burns Ward and their ever-present full-time companion, 'Rusty Nails'

Robert P (called Pete) and Aileen Rumball.

Were the first couple to be married in the John Flynn Memorial Church in Alice Springs in 1956, and are still going strong (?) at the time of writing, early 2014.

They both have a long family, as well as personal, history in "The Territory", (Northern Territory, Australia)

Aileen is the only daughter of the late Alex McLeod of Utopia Station (now known as Urapuntja), educated at PGC in Adelaide, and at the time of their engagement was a radio operator for the Royal Flying Doctor Base in the Alice.

Pete was the only son of Bob Rumball, one of the first people to regularly travel the track to the Alice from the Southern Flinders Ranges as a representative for the Shell Company of Australia. Bob eventually moved to the Alice and Pete was educated at Queens College in Adelaide.

Bob took over the Shell Depot in the Alice as an agency and Pete joined him in this business, also taking on other agencies including Southern Cross Machinery. (windmills, diesel engines, pumps etc.)

After many years Pete and Aileen ended up in Queensland, where they operated two Motor Bike shops.

While running the Motor Bike shops Pete suffered a 60% burns accident which put him in the Royal Brisbane Hospital Burns Ward for three months, followed by twelve month convalescence.

On retirement they sold up everything, bought a nine metre caravan and travelled around the goldfields of NSW, Victoria and West Australia, prospecting for Gold with considerable success.

This was the time that Rusty Nails joined them as a puppy, and his exploits in the goldfields have been the subject of several books by Pete Rumball. (Rusty Nails in the Goldfields) At Amazon, both Paper-Back and Kindle eBook.

All three are now in a Brisbane retirement village and Pete spends his time writing articles and books, and being woken by Rusty every morning at 4.00am to go prospecting.

www.ingramcontent.com/pod-product-compliance
Lightning Source LLC
Chambersburg PA
CBHW040819200526
45159CB00024B/3052